spot light on spinal anesthesia hypotension

Hala Mostafa Goma, MD, Professor of anesthesia, Faculty of medicine Cairo University.

Table of contents

Introduction: 4
Anatomical considerations 7
Autonomic supply 18

Effects of local anesthetics 21
Autonomic blockade 22
Effects pharmacological sympathetictomy 27
Factors affect degree of decline blood pressure 29
Spinal anesthesia induced Hypotension in pregnant women 30
Structure of placenta 30
Effects of change in systemic vascular resistance on uterine blood flow: 33
Effect of uterine contractions on placental blood flow 34
Spinal induced hypotension and the intrauterine fetus 36
Preoperative evaluation 37
Pharmacological management for spinal induced hypotension 39
PHARMACOLOGY OF LOCAL ANESTHETICS 40

Role of intravenous fluids in protection against spinal induced hypotension *52*

Crystalloid versus colloid in spinal induced hypotension: *59*

Drugs used in spinal induced hypotension(epinephrine and phenylepherine). *61*

Ephedrine *62*

Ondansetron **71**

Role of pharmacologic agents in **prevention of hypotension:** *73*

Role of onandestron in spinal induced hypotension **75**

References **77**

1-Introduction:

- The anesthetic of certain surgery take into account the well-being of patients: the surgent ,and anesthesiologist.
- General anesthesia is associated with higher mortality rate in comparison to regional anesthesia
- Spinal anesthesia provides a fast, intense, and symmetrical sensory and motor block of high quality in patients undergoing lower abdominal and lower limb surgeries. Spinal anesthesia has fewer sides' effects and risk than general anesthesia .patients recovers faster and can go home sooner.
- Spinal anesthesia is used for genital, urinary tract, or lower body procedures. A successful regional anesthesia effectively suppress many of pain mediated stress response ,it block release of stress hormones as adrenaline , nor adrenaline ,cortical .These three hormones cause increase in blood pressure , heart rate and increase in plasma glucose. Spinal anesthesia is also associated with lesser amount of surgical hemorrhage .spinal anesthesia produces few adverse effects on respiratory system as high spinal block is avoided. so it is better in controlling air way, and there is less risk of air way obstruction or aspiration of gastric contents. Spinal anesthesia provides excellent muscle relaxation for lower abdominal and lower limb surgery.post

operative deep vein thrombosis, and pulmonary embolism are less common following spinal anesthesia.

- Hypotension during spinal anesthesia is the most common complication of spinal anesthesia. Hypotension is due to sympathetic nervous system blockade. As a result, decreased systemic vascular resistance and peripheral pooling of blood occurs which decreases cardiac output.

- So a spinal block will temporarily block the sympathetic transmission at the affected levels, leading to vasodilatation and loss of sweating in the affected dermatomes. if the block is allowed to spread to levels supplying cardiac sympathetic fibers(T1-T4),there will be loss of inotropic and chronotropic drive to the heart and progressive hypotension. the parasympathetic supply to the heart coming from the vagus nerve will be unaffected by the spinal block, leading to unopposed parasympathetic stimulation and bradycardia spinal induced hypotension can cause significant morbidity and mortality, it may be associated with severe nausea and vomiting ,aspiration if there is loss of consciousness.

- Hypotension during caesarean section under spinal anaesthesia is very frequent. and if not prevented, it can induce complication for the mother and/ or the fetus. Untreated, severe hypotension leads to serious risks to both mother (unconsciousness, pulmonary aspiration, apnoea or even cardiac arrest) and baby (impaired placental perfusion leading to hypoxia, fetal acidosis and neurological injury).

- Prevention and treatment of spinal induced hypotension can be by either intravenous preload or pharmacological drugs.
- Fluid can be crystalloids or colloids.
- Drugs as Ephedrine, Epinephrine ,phenyl Epherine ondansetron .Ephedrine is a non-catecholamine sympathomimetic agent that stimulates alpha and beta adrenergic receptors directly and predominantly indirectly, producing its effects by releasing norepinephrine from sympathetic nerve endings
- Role of ondansetron in spinal induced hypotension:

Serotonin in response to decreased blood volume activates Chemoreceptors . Serotonin is released from activated thrombocytes. Serotonin Activate 5-HT3 receptors, which are G protein coupled, ligand-gated fast-ion channels, results in increased efferent vagal nerve activity, frequently producing bradycardia . Mechanoreceptors in the heart wall that trigger the BJR, participate in systemic responses to hyper- and hypo-volaemia. In response to hypovolaemia, stimulation of cardiac sensory receptors in the left ventricle induces the BJR and results in reflex bradycardia, vasodilation and hypotension.

2-Anatomical considerations

2-1 The vertebral column

The spine is composed of the vertebral bones and fibro cartilaginous intervertebral disks. There are 7 cervical, 12 thoracic, and 5 lumbar vertebrae. The sacrum is a fusion of 5 sacral vertebrae, and there are small rudimentary coccygeal vertebrae. The spine as a whole provides structural support for the body and protection for the spinal cord and nerves, and allows a degree of mobility in several spatial planes. At each vertebral level, paired spinal nerves exit the central nervous system.

The lumbar vertebrae have a large anterior cylindrical vertebral body. A hollow ring is defined anteriorly by the vertebral body, laterally by the pedicles and transverse processes, and posteriorly by the laminae and spinous processes. The laminae extend between the transverse processes and the spinous processes and the pedicle extends between the vertebral body and the transverse processes. When stacked vertically, the hollow rings become the spinal canal in which the spinal cord and its coverings sit. The individual vertebral bodies are connected by the intervertebral disks.

There are four small synovial joints at each vertebra, two articulating with the vertebra above it and two with the vertebra below. These are the facet joints, which are adjacent to the transverse processes.

The pedicles are notched superiorly and inferiorly, these notches forming the intervertebral foramina, from which the spinal nerves exit.

The vertebral column usually contains three curves. The cervical and lumbar curves are convex anteriorly, and the thoracic curve is convex posteriorly. The vertebral column curves, along with gravity, baricity of local anesthetic, and patient position, influence the spread of local anesthetics in the subarachnoid space Ligamentous elements provide structural support and together with supporting muscles help maintain the unique shape. Ventrally, the vertebral bodies and intervertebral discs are connected and supported by the anterior and posterior longitudinal ligaments. Dorsally, the ligamentumflavum, interspinous ligament, and supraspinous ligament provide additional stability

2-2 The spinal canal

The spinal canal contains the spinal cord with its coverings (the meninges), spinal nerves, fatty tissue, and a venous plexus.

2-3.The meninges

The meninges are composed of three layers from within outward: the pia mater, the arachnoid mater, and the dura mater; all are continuous with their cranial counterparts. The pia mater is closely adherent to the spinal cord, whereas the arachnoid mater is usually closely adherent to the thicker and denser dura mater. Cerebrospinal fluid (CSF) is contained between the pia and arachnoid maters in the subarachnoid space. The spinal subdural space is generally a poorly demarcated, potential space that exists between the dura and arachnoid membranes. The epidural space is a better defined potential space within the spinal canal that is bounded by the dura and the ligamentumflavum. The dural sac and the subarachnoid and subdural spaces usually extend to S2 in adults and often to S3 in children .

2-4 Cerebrospinal fluid (CSF)

Cerebrospinal fluid supports and protects the brain and the spinal cord. The total volume in adults is about 130 ml and the average daily production is 500 ml. Spinal CSF accounts for only 35 ml of the total volume. Although some may drain into local venous plexuses, most returns to the cranium for drainage.

2-5 The spinal cord

The spinal cord forms the elongated, nearly cylindrical part of the central nervous system (CNS). The length of the spinal cord varies according to age. In the first trimester, the spinal cord extends to the end of the spinal column, but as the fetus ages, the vertebral column lengthens more than the spinal cord. At birth, the spinal cord ends at approximately L3 and in the adult, the cord ends at approximately L1 with 30% of people having a cord that ends at T12 and 10% at L3 [60].i A sacral spinal cord in an adult has been reported, though this is extremely rare. The length of the spinal cord must always be kept in mind when neuraxial anesthesia is performed, as injection into the cord can cause great damage and result in paralysis.

2-6 Spinal nerves

Thirty one pairs of spinal nerves arise from the spinal cord, each nerve having a ventral and a dorsal root, the latter being distinguished by the presence of an oval swelling; the spinal ganglion which contain numerous nerve cells. As the sensory fibers traverse the posterior aspect of the subarachnoid space, they tend to lay dependent in a
supine patient, thus making them particularly vulnerable to hyperbaric solutions containing local anesthetic. At the cervical level, the nerves arise above their respective vertebrae, but starting at T1 they exit below their vertebrae. As a result, there are eight cervical nerve roots but only seven cervical vertebrae. The cervical and upper thoracic nerve roots emerge from the spinal cord and exit the vertebral foramina nearly at the same level . But because the spinal cord normally ends at L1, lower nerve roots course some distance before exiting the intervertebral foramina.

These lower spinal nerves form the caudaequina. Therefore, performing a lumbar (subarachnoid) puncture below L1 in an adult (L3 in a child) avoids potential needle trauma to the cord; damage to the caudaequina is unlikely as these nerve roots float in the dural sac below L1 and tend to be pushed away (rather than pierced) by an advancing needle .

When performing spinal anesthesia using the midline approach, the layers of anatomy that are traversed (from posterior to anterior) are skin, subcutaneous fat, supraspinous ligament, interspinous ligament, ligamentumflavum, dura mater, subdural space, arachnoid mater, and finally the subarachnoid space.When the paramedian technique is applied, the spinal needle should traverse the skin, subcutaneous fat, ligamentumflavum, dura mater, subdural space, arachnoid mater, and then pass into the subarachnoid space.

2-7 Surface Anatomy

When preparing for spinal anesthetic blockade, it is important to find landmarks on the patient. The iliac crests usually mark the interspace between the fourth and fifth lumbar vertebrae, and a line can be drawn between them to help locate this interspace (Tuffier's line).

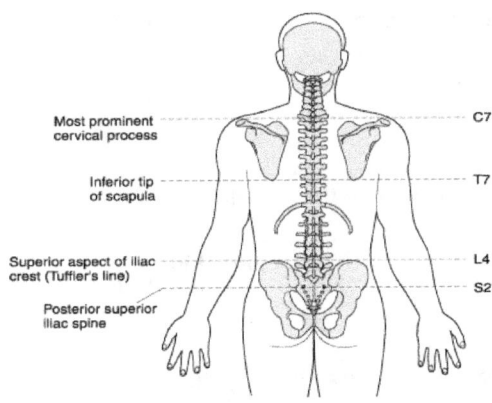

Figure 1 surface landmarks for identifying spinal levels.

Care must be taken to feel for the soft area between the spinous processes to locate the interspace. Depending on the level of anesthesia necessary for the surgery and the ability to feel for the interspace, the L3-4 interspace or the L4-5 interspace can be used to introduce the spinal needle. Because the spinal cord ends at the L1 to L2 level, it would not be wise to attempt spinal anesthesia at or above this level

Procedure	Dermatomal Level
Upper abdominal surgery	T4
Intestinal, gynecologic, and urologic surgery	T6
Transurethral resection of the prostate	T10
Vaginal delivery of a fetus, and hip surgery	T10
Thigh surgery and lower leg amputations	L1
Foot and ankle surgery	L2
Perineal and anal surgery	S2 to S5 (saddle block)

Table 1: Spinal Anesthesia dermatomal Levels of for some Surgical Procedures

.

A dermatome is an area of skin innervated by sensory fibers from a single spinal nerve. The tenth thoracic (T10) dermatome corresponds to the umbilicus, the sixth thoracic (T6) dermatome the xiphoid, and the fourth thoracic (T4) dermatome the nipples .To achieve surgical anaesthesia for a given procedure, the extent of spinal anaesthesia must reach a certain dermatomal level.

figure 2 Surface dermatomal supply.

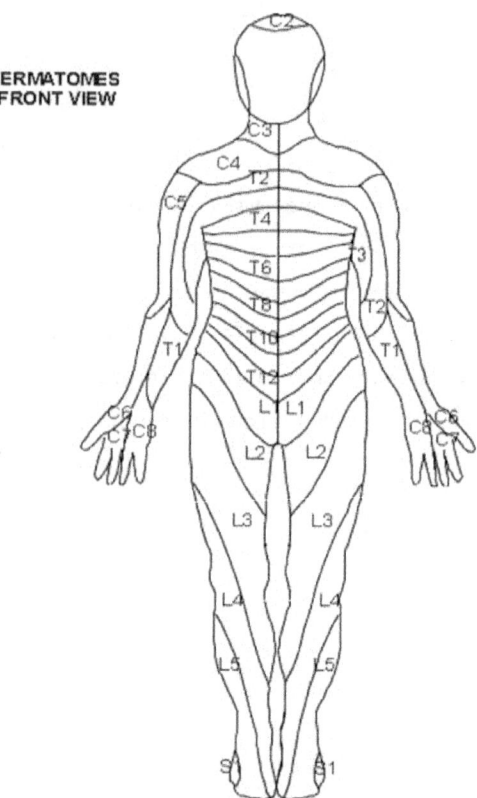

The spinal canal contains the spinal cord with its coverings (the meninges), fatty tissue, and a venous plexus. The meninges are composed of three layers: the pia mater, the arachnoid mater, and the dura mater; all are contiguous with their cranial counterparts. The pia mater is closely adherent to the spinal cord, whereas the arachnoid mater is usually closely adherent to the thicker and denser dura mater CSF is an isotonic, aqueous medium with a constitution similar to interstitial fluid. CSF is contained between the pia and arachnoid matters in the subarachnoid space.

Spinal cord normally extends from the foramen magnum to the level of L_1 in adults. The anterior and posterior nerve roots at each spinal level join one another and exit the intervertebral foramina forming spinal nerves from C_1 to S_5. At the cervical level, the nerves arise above their respective vertebrae, but starting at T_1 they exit below their vertebrae. Because the spinal cord normally ends at L_1, lower nerve roots course some distance before exiting the intervertebral

2-8 Autonomic supply:

It is purely efferent neuron system(preganglionic and post ganglionic fibers.it arises from discreteparts of CNS

1-only 4 cranial nerve contain autonomic fibers

III cranial nerve (occulomotor nerve).

VI cranial nerve (facial nerve).

IX cranial nerve (Glossopharngeal nerve).

X cranial nerve (Vagus Nerve).

2-all12 thoracic segments.

3-all upper Lumber segments.

4-2,3,4 sacral segments.

It was found that thoracic and lumber parts have complementary functions,while the cranial and sacral parts have complementary functionsbut both are antagonistic.for example the vagus nerve supplies the GIT till the transverse colon , while the sacral autonomic supplies the rest of GITboth do the same function ,it is motorto the wall,and inhibitoryto the sphincters.greater and lesser splanchnic nerve arise from thoracic and lumber parts supplythe

GIT produce the opposite function (relaxation of the wall,and contraction of the sphincters.

The autonomic nervous systemcan be divided into

Thoracolumber or sympathetic nervous system.

Craniosacral or parasympathetic nervous system.

Autonomic ganglion:

They are collection of nerve cells present outside CNS.autonomic ganglia are the seat of rely of preganglionic fibers may rely on so many postganglionic fibers . the ratio between the pregagnlionic to post ganlionicfibers in sympathetic chain may be 1:8030.

Sympathetic system relays mainly in the lateral sympathetic chain and some fibers relay in collateral ganglia.

The preganglionic sympathetic supply to the lower limb is originated from neurones in the lateral horn of the lower thoracic (T10, T11 and T12) and upper lumbar (L1, L2) spinal cord segments. Fibres pass in white rami to the sympathetic chain, and synapse in the lumbar and sacral ganglia. Postganglionic fibres pass in grey rami to enter the lumbar and sacral plexuses, and many are distributed via the cutaneous branches of the nerves derived from these plexuses. The blood vessels to the lower limb receive their sympathetic supply by adjacent peripheral nerves. Postganglionic fibres pass with the iliac arteries supply the pelvis but may supply vessels in the upper thigh also.

3-Effects of local anesthetics:

Local anesthetics placed in the subarachnoid space will block sensory, autonomic, and motor impulses by their action on anterior/posterior spinal nerve roots, and the dorsal root ganglion when they pass through the CSF.

3-1 *Blockade of the anterior nerve root fibers.*

It will blocke the efferent motor and autonomic transmission.
Blockade of posterior nerve root fibers.

3-2 Autonomic Blockade:

Class	Action	Myelin	Size
Aα	Motor	Yes	++++
Aβ	Light touch, pressure pain	Yes	+++
Aγ	Proprioception	Yes	+++
Aδ	Pain, temperature	Yes	++
B	Preganglionic sympathetic fibers	Yes	++
C	Pain, pressure	No	+

Physiological considerations are determined by the effects of interrupting the afferent and efferent innervations of somatic and visceral structures. Somatic structures are traditionally related with sensory and motor innervations, while the visceral structures are more related to the autonomic nervous system.

Prevention of pain and skeletal muscle relaxation are classic objectives of central blockade. Nerve fibers are not homogenous. There are three main types of nerve fibers designated A, B and C. The A group has four sub-groups alpha, beta, gamma and delta. The minimum concentration of local anesthetic required to stop transmission (Cm) varies depending upon fiber size.

Most of the visceral effects of central blockade are mediated by interruption of autonomic impulses to various organ systems. Sympathetic blockade results in cardiovascular changes of hemodynamic consequence in proportion to the degree of sympathectomy. The sympathetic chain originates from the lumbar and thoracic spinal cord. The fibres involved in smooth muscle tone of the arterial and venous circulation arise from T_5 and L_1. Arteries retain most of their tone despite sympathectomy because of local mediators and there is no arteriolar vasoplegia, but the venous circulation does not. The consequence of total sympathectomy is an increase in the volume of the capacitance vessels, specially in the splanchnic circulation, decreasing the venous return to the heart and hypotension occurs.

The cardiac accelerator fibers are sympathetic efferents, which increase heart rate when stimulated. When blocked by high central l blockade, unopposed vagal action leads to bradycardia.

Prophylactic administration of pharmacologic agents may be more effective than prehydration to prevent hypotension. α-adrenergic agents (e.g., phenylephrine) reliably increase arterial blood pressure by increasing systemic vascular resistance, however, heart rate and cardiac output may decrease because of increased after load. α- and β- adrenergic agonists (e.g., ephedrine) are effective for increasing arterial blood pressure preventing hypotension but act by primarily increasing heart rate and cardiac output with a smaller increase in systemic vascular resistance .Initial treatment can be tailored to α-agonists on patients with hypotension and mixed α and β agonist on patients with both hypotension and bradycardia.

Clinically significant alterations in pulmonary physiology are usually minimal with neuroaxial blockade because the diaphragm is innervated by the phrenic nerve with fibers originating from C_3-C_5. Even with high levels, tidal volume is unchanged; there is only a decrease in vital capacity, which results from a loss of abdominal muscles' contribution to forced expiration.

Patients with severe chronic lung disease may rely upon accessory muscles of respiration (intercostal and abdominal muscles) to actively inspire or exhale. High levels of neural blockade will impair these muscles. Similarly, effective coughing and clearing of secretions require these muscles for expiration. For these reasons, neuroaxial blocks should be used with caution in patients with limited respiratory reserve .

Sympathetic block occurs before sensory, followed by motor.

4-Effects of pharmacological sympathetictomy :

4-1 Cardiovascular Effects:

1-Decrease in blood pressure (33% incidence of hypotension in non-obstetric populations)

2-Decrease in heart rate (13% incidence of bradycardia

3-Decrease in cardiac contractility

<u>4-2 Risk factors for bradycardia during spinal anesthesia:</u>

1-patients with a baseline heart rate of less than 60

2- ASA I .

3-prolonged P-R interval

4- Beta blocker administrationa .

<u>4-3 Risk factors for hypotension include</u>

   1- age more 40 years

   2- a baseline SBP more120 mmHg.

   3- a lumbar

   4- puncture at or above L2-L3

5-Sympathectomy:

Nerve fibers that affect vasomotor tone of the arterial, and venous vessels arise from T5-L1.

1- it decreases right atrial filling results in decreased stimulation of the intrinsic chronotropic stretch receptors. this will lead to decrease heart rate.

2- Decreased SVR (systemic vascular resistance).

5-1 Level of sympathetic block:

The sympathetic dermatome ranges from 2-6 levels higher than the sensory dermatome level.

Sympathectomy is directly related to the height of the block and results in venous and arterial vasodilatation. Dilation of the venous system is mainely responsible for reduction in blood pressure because the arterial system controls its vascular tone.

Pooling of blood in the venous system because it contains about 75% of the total blood volume, while the arterial system contains about 25%.

Total peripheral vascular resistance in the normal patient (normal cardiac output and normovolemic) will decrease 15-18%. In the elderly the systemic vascular resistance may decrease as much as 25%

5-2 Heart rate

It decreases during a high block due to blockade of the cardioaccelerator fibers (T1-T4). Heart rate may also decline as a result of a decrease in SVR, decreased right atrial filling, and decreases in the intrinsic chronotropic stretch receptor response.

5-3 Risk factors for hypotension in non obstetric patients:

1- Block height T5 or more.
2- Age 40 years. or more.
3- Baseline systolic blood pressure less than 120 mmHg.
4- Spinal puncture above L3–L4.

5-4 Factors affect degree of decline blood pressure in parturient:

1-age

2-co-existing diseases (i.e. cardiovascular disease, renal dysfunction, etc.).

3-Base line systolic pressure.

4=head up position.

5-the weight of a gravid uterus on venous return in the parturient may cause further declines in blood pressure.

6-sudden cardiac arrest may be seen with spinal anesthesia due to unopposed vagal stimulation.

5-6 Mechanism of hypotension:

The factors responsible for the vasodilatation:

1. Decreased vascular responsiveness to the pressor effects of angiotensin II and norepinephrine.
2. Increased endothelial prostacycline.
3. Enhanced nitric oxide production
4. Ortic stiffness.

8-Structure of placenta:

The placenta is composed of both maternal and fetal tissues that consist of a basal and a chorionic plate it can be appeared as a semi permeable membrane that provides a communication between maternal and fetal circulation.

The intervillous space separates the plates and is subdivided by decidual tissue. Chorionic villi and spiral arteries protrude into this intervillous space. About 80% of the uterine blood flow passes through the intervillous space. Placental transfer from the mother to the fetus occurs when maternal blood flows into the intervillous space from the spiral artery.

40% to 50% of fetal cardiac output goes to the placenta, and a similar amount returns to the heart through the umbilical vein. Fetal blood enters the placenta through the two umbilical arteries, which arise from the internal iliac arteries. These arteries subdivide and eventually form umbilical capillaries that traverse the chorionic villi.

8-1 umbilical-placental circulation

The umbilical-placental circulation is regulated
1-physiologic reflex changes
2-neuroendocrine axis.

Numerous substances, including prostaglandins, endorphins, catecholamines, and vasopressin, all play roles in umbilical-placental microcirculation.

8-2 Placental Blood Flow:

placental blood flow is an important determinant of fetal oxygen and nutrient supply .The transport across the placenta allows respiratory gases ,and many solutes to reach equal concentration between the maternal intervillous space blood and fetal capillary blood.

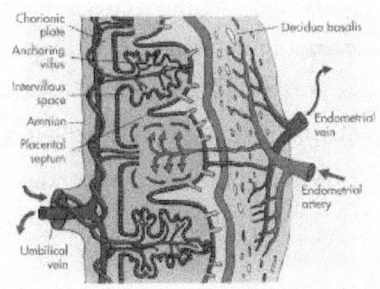

anatomical structure of the placenta

8-3 Uterine blood flow

Uterine blood flow increases more than 50 times above non pregnant values. nearly 90% of total uterine blood flow near term received by placenta , only 10% supply myometrium, and endometrium .

ther is doubling of maternal cardiac, and a 40% increase in blood volume. factors increase the uterine blood flow are placental growth, and maternal arterial vasodilation.

Placental intervillous space volume almost triples between weeks 22 and 36 of gestation. so there is increase in placental diffusing capacity. direct estrogen-induced vasodilation will increase the blood flow . This effect is mediated through the release of a number of local vasodilatory agents contribute to this effect including prostanoids (PGI_2), nitric oxide, and kinins. These combined effects provide uterine blood flow rates at term of at least 750 mL/min, or 10% to 15% of maternal cardiac output. A gradual return to the prepregnancy blood volume occurs at 6 to 9 weeks post partum.

8-4 Effects of change in systemic vascular resistance on uterine blood flow:

Vasodilation:
Systemically administered vasodilator agents preferentially dilate systemic vessels, reducing uterine blood flow.
1- antihypertensive agents
2- regional anesthesia with sympathetic blockade

Vasoconstriction:
1- pressor agent–induced increases in uterine vascular resistance may exceed increases in systemic vascular resistance, reducing uteroplacental blood flow.

1- increased maternal plasma catecholamine levels during preeclampsia.

2- pressor agents administered for treatment of maternal hypotension may have adverse effects on uterine blood flow.

3- Although respiratory gases are important regulators of blood flow in a number of organs, there is no indication that either oxygen or carbon dioxide are responsible for short-term changes in uterine blood flow.

8-5 Effect of uterine contractions on placental blood flow:

During uterine contractions the relationship between uterine arterial and venous pressures and blood flow no longer holds. Since intrauterine pressures are directly transmitted to the intervillous space, increases in intrauterine pressure are reflected by decreases in placental blood flow.

8-6 Other agents affect utroplacental blood flow
Calcitonin gene–related peptide produces uterine artery relaxation and enhances uterine artery blood flow and improved fetal growth. Phosphodiesterase 5–specific inhibitors, including sildenafil, tadalafil, and vardenafil, enhance nitric oxide's vasodilatory effect by inhibition of cGMP (second messenger in the nitric oxide cascade) breakdown, with resultant relaxation of vascular smooth muscle.

8-9 Umbilical blood flow

Fetal blood flow to the umbilical circulation represents approximately 40% of the combined output of both fetal ventricles Over the last third of gestation, increases in umbilical blood flow are proportional to fetal growth, so that umbilical blood flow remains constant when normalized to fetal weight. Human umbilical venous flow can be estimated through the use of triplex mode ultrasonography. Although increases in villous capillary number represent the primary contributor to gestation-dependent increases in umbilical blood flow, the factors that regulate this change are not known.

Short-term changes in umbilical blood flow are primarily regulated by perfusion pressure. The relationship between flow and perfusion pressure is linear in the umbilical circulation. As a result, small (2 to 3 mm Hg) increases in umbilical vein pressure evoke proportional decreases in umbilical blood flow. Because both the umbilical artery and vein are enclosed in the amniotic cavity, pressure changes caused by increases in uterine tone are transmitted equally to these vessels without changes in umbilical blood flow. Relative to the uteroplacental bed, the fetoplacental circulation is resistant to vasoconstrictive effects of infused pressor agents, and umbilical blood flow is preserved unless cardiac output decreases. Thus, despite catecholamine-induced changes in blood flow is distribution, and increases in blood pressure during acute hypoxia, umbilical blood flow is maintained over a relatively wide range of oxygen tensions. Endogenous vasoactive autacoids have been identified; nitric oxide may also be important. Endothelin-1, in particular, is associated with diminished Fetoplacental blood flow.

8-10 Spinal induced hypotension and the intrauterine fetus:

Adequate intravillous space blood flow and oxygenation are probably related to normal differential intra myometrial ,and maternal blood pressure and enough relaxation in between uterine contractions, during maternal hypotension there is fetal brady cardia similar to bradycardia due to uterine contractions, the ECG pattern is U shaped ,and then longer U shaped ECG with irregular pattern indicates the presence of fetal hypoxia.

Management of hypotension due to subarachnoid blockade:

1-patient's cardiac function and medical history should be taken into account prior to this measure.

2- Using a proper "dose" of local anesthetics is crucial.

3- Volume loading the patient with 10-20 ml/kg of crystalloid fluid or appropriate amount of colloid immediately prior and during the administration of a spinal anesthetic may be helpful.

4-The Left uterine displacement is essential for the parturient.

5-Trendelenburg position may increase blood pressure by autotransfusion.

6-Bradycardia should be rapidly treated with atropine (0.5 – 1 mg IVP).

9-Preoperative evaluation:
9-1 history suggestive hypotension:
Symptoms suggestive of cardiovascular disease at term:
Shortness of breath,
Palpitations,
Dizziness,
Edema,
Poor exercise tolerance.
Chest pain,
Syncope,
Severe arrhythmias,

9-2 Physical examination of the term pregnant woman :
auscultation commonly revealing a wide, loud, split first heart sound, an S3 sound, and a soft systolic ejection murmur. systolic murmur more than grade 3, or diastolic murmur suggest severe disease and warrant further investigation.

9-3 Investigations:
1. electrocardiogram,
Chest radiograph.

2-echocardiogram.

9-4 Prophylactic measures against supine hypotension:

In the operating room, a small pillow or "wedge" should be used to provide left uterine displacement of 15 to 20 degrees.

9-5 Management of hypotension due to subarachnoid blockade:

1-patient's cardiac function and medical history should be taken into account prior to this measure.

2- Using a proper "dose" of local anesthetics is crucial.

3- Volume loading the patient with 10-20 ml/kg of crystalloid fluid or appropriate amount of colloid immediately prior and during the administration of a spinal anesthetic may be helpful.

4-The Left uterine displacement is essential for the parturient.

5-Trendelenburg position may increase blood pressure by auto transfusion.

6-Bradycardia should be rapidly treated with atropine (0.5 – 1 mg IVP).

10- Pharmacological management for spinal induced hypotension:

Three pharmacological factors involved in the management of spinal induced hypotension:

1-local anesthetic dose and its toxicity (pubivacaine).

2-pre hyderation fluids:

 a- Crystalloids (lactated Ringer solution).

 B -colloids (Hest solution,albumin).

3-Drugs:

 1- Epinephrine.

 2-phenylepherine.

 3-Ephedrine

   4- ondansetron.

11- PHARMACOLOGY OF LOCAL ANESTHETICS

11-1 Bupivicaine structure:

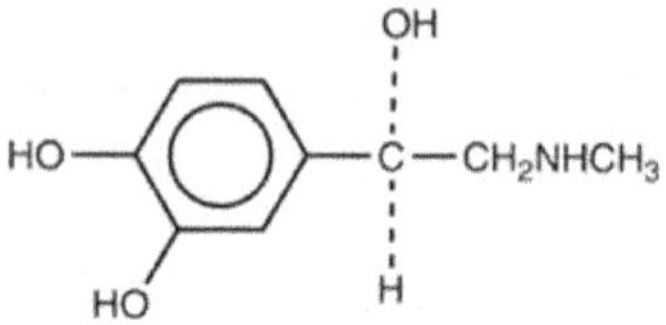

Figure 3 : Pharmacologic structure of bupivacain

Most local anesthetic agents consist of a lipophilic group (aromatic benzene ring) connected by an intermediate chain via an ester or amide linkage to an ionizable group (e.g., a tertiary amine). Local anesthetics may therefore be classified as aminoester or aminoamide compounds. The amino-ester local anesthetics are: procaine, chlorprocaine and tetracaine. The amino-amides consist of lidocaine, mepivacaine, prilocaine, bupivacaine, and etidocaine. The ester and amide local anesthetics differ in their chemical stability, biotransformation, and allergic potential. Amides are extremely stable agents, while esters are relatively unstable in solution.

Local anesthetics are weak bases and are made available clinically as salts to increase their solubility and stability. Inside the body they exist as the uncharged base (unionized form) or as a cation (ionized form). The relative proportions of these two forms is governed by the pKa specific for each local anesthetic and the pH of the body fluids, pKa of bupivacaine is 8.1

11-2 Mechanism of Action of Bupivicaine:

The primary mechanism of action of bupivacaine is blockage of voltage-gated sodium channels. The excitable membrane of nerve axons like the membrane of cardiac muscle fibers and neuronal cell bodies maintains a resting membrane potential of -90 to -60 mV. During excitation the sodium channels open, and fast inward sodium current quickly depolarizes the membrane towards the sodium equilibrium potential (+40 mV). As a result of depolarization, the sodium channels close (inactivate) and potassium channels open. The outward flow of potassium repolarizes the membrane towards the potassium equilibrium potential (about -90 mV) repolarization returns the membrane to the resting state. The trans-membrane ionic gradients are maintained by the sodium pump.

Thus, there appears to be a single binding site for local anesthetics on the sodium channel. Sodium currents are reduced by local anesthetics because the drug-bound channels fail to open. Inactivation and anesthetic binding prevent the conformational changes that constitute the activation process by fully or partially immobilizing the channel. Pain impulses fail to traverse the drugged axon. Impulse activity entering the anesthetized region thus maintains its own failure

11-3 Pharmacokinetics:

The onset of sensory blockade following spinal block with bupivacaine is very rapid (within one minute); maximum motor blockade and maximum dermatome level are achieved within 15 minutes in most cases. Duration of sensory blockade (time to return of complete sensation in the operative site or regression of two dermatomes) averages 2 hours with or without 0.2 mg epinephrine. The time to return of complete motor ability averages 3.5 hours without the addition of epinephrine and 4.5 hours if 0.2 mg epinephrine is added.

- *Absorption:*

The systemic absorption of local anesthetics is determined by the site of injection, dosage, addition of vasoconstrictor agent, and pharmacologic profile of the agent itself. The maximum blood level of local anesthetic is related to the total dose of drug administered for any particular site of administration

- *Distribution:*

Local anesthetics are distributed throughout all body tissues, but the relative concentration in different tissues varies. In general the more highly perfused organs show higher concentrations of local anesthetic drug than the less well perfused organs. In particular these agents are rapidly extracted by lung tissue, so that the whole blood level of local anesthetics decreases markedly as they pass through the pulmonary vasculature. The highest percentage of an injected dose of local anesthetic is found in skeletal muscle

- *Biotransformation and Excretion:*

Bupivacaine is metabolized in the liver via conjugation with glucuronic acid. The excretion of bupivacaine occurs via the kidney. Less than 5% of the unchanged drug is excreted via the kidney into the urine. The major proportion of the injected agent appears in the urine in the form of various metabolites.

11-4 Mechanisms of intrathecal drug spread:

The CSF of the vertebral canal occupies a narrow space (2-3 mm deep) surrounding the spinal cord and caudaequina enclosed by the arachnoid mater. As the local anesthetic solution is injected, it will spread initially by displacement of CSF.

The next stage which may be the most crucial, is spread due to the interplay between the densities of both CSF and local anesthetic solution under influence of gravity. Gravity will be 'applied' through patients' position (supine, sitting, etc...)

11-5 Factors affecting intrathecal spread:

1- Characteristics of the injected solution:

Baricity:

Most plain solutions exhibit greater variability to effect and are less predictable, that the block may either be too low, and the block inadequate for surgery, or excessively high causing side effects

Hyperbaric solutions are more predictable, with greater spread in the direction of gravity.

2-Volume/ dose/ concentration injected:

Clearly, it is impossible to change one of these factors without changing the other, but this is not always appreciated. Volume is an important determinant of the spread of isobaric solution. A change in dose will be accompanied by a change in either volume or concentration.

3-Temperature of the solution:

Both CSF and local anesthetics exhibit a decrease in density with increasing temperature

4-Viscosity:

Addition of glucose to aqueous solution increases viscosity as well as density.

11-6 Local anesthetic drugs and additives:

Studies of a wide range of local anesthetic drugs indicate that intrathecal spread is the same, no matter which one is used, as long as the other factors are controlled. Solutions containing vasoconstrictors spread in exactly the same way as those without, although block duration may be prolonged. Alkalinization of the solution does not increase spread, but does prolong duration

The addition of other drugs, such as opioids or midazolam, has a dual effect. First, such additions are achieved by mixing the adjuvant and local anesthetic solutions, usually reducing the density of the latter. In theory this might make the mixture behave in a more hypobaric manner, but no effect has been shown in clinical practice, suggesting that the changes in density are small. The second effect is seen with opioids, which increase mean spread and delay regression, but opioids do so no matter what the route of administration either intrathecal or I.V. Presumably, this is pharmacological enhancement of subclinical block at the limits of the local anesthetic's spread through the CSF.

11-7 Advantages of local anesthetic neural blockade include:

Adequate anesthesia plus postoperative relief of pain with reduced requirements for systemic opioids resulting in avoidance of sedation and respiratory depression. More importantly, the inhibition of the neuroendocrinal response to surgery, trauma induced nociceptive impulses, and blunting of the autonomic and somatic responses to pain facilitate breathing, coughing, sighing and early ambulation. This results in restoration of pulmonary function and reduction of post operative chest infection and pulmonary collapse. Finally, efferent sympathetic blockade results in increased blood flow to the region of neural blockade resulting in better wound healing and reduced risk of deep venous thrombosis and thromboembolism.

11-8 Toxicity:

Systemic reactions to local anesthetics involve primarily the central nervous system (CNS) and the cardiovascular system. In general the CNS is more susceptible to the systemic actions of local anesthetic agents than the cardiovascular system. The dose and blood level of local anesthetic required to produce CNS toxicity is usually lower than that which results in circulatory collapse.

- *Central Nervous System Toxicity*

The initial symptoms of local anesthetic-induced CNS toxicity involve feelings of lightheadedness and dizziness followed frequently by visual and auditory disturbances such as difficulty in focusing and tinnitus. Other subjective CNS symptoms include disorientation and occasional feelings of drowsiness. Objective signs of CNS toxicity are usually excitatory motor in nature and include shivering, muscular twitching, and tremors initially involving muscles of the face and distal parts of the extremities. Ultimately generalized convulsions of a tonic-clonic nature occur. If a sufficiently large dose or a rapid intravenous injection is administered the initial signs of CNS excitation are rapidly followed by a state of generalized CNS depression.

- *Cardiovascular System Toxicity*

Local anesthetic agents can exert a direct action both on the heart and peripheral blood vessels. The primary cardiac electrophysiological effect of local anesthetics is a decrease in the maximum rate of depolarization in Purkinje fibers and ventricular muscle. This reduction in the maximum rate of depolarization is believed to be due to a decrease in the availability of fast sodium channels in cardiac membranes

Local anesthetic drugs also exert a dose dependent negative inotropic action on the heart. The more potent agents as bupivacaine depress cardiac contractility at the lowest concentrations Local anesthetics exert a biphasic effect on peripheral vascular smooth muscle. Low concentrations of bupivacaine produce vasoconstriction, while high concentrations increase arteriolar diameter.

The cardiotoxicity of bupivacaine appears to differ from that of other local anesthetics in the following manner:

a) The dosage required for irreversible cardiovascular collapse is lower for bupivacaine than for other local anesthetic agents.

b) Ventricular arrhythmias and fatal ventricular fibrillation may occur following rapid intravenous administration of a large dose of bupivacaine. The arrhythmogenic action of bupivacaine may be related to an inhibition of the fast sodium channels in the cardiac membrane.

c) Pregnant patients may be more sensitive to the cardiotoxic effects of bupivacaine than non-pregnant patients

The maximum safe dose of bupivacaine is 3 mg/kg. However, inadvertent intravascular injection is the most common cause of local anesthetic toxicity even if anesthetic was administered within the recommended dose range

11-9 *Allergic Reactions*

The aminoester agents may produce allergic-type reactions since these agents are derivatives of para-aminobenzoic acid which is known to be allergic.

The amide local anesthetics are not derivatives of para-aminobenzoic acid and allergic reactions to them are extremely rare.

11-10 Management of Local Anesthetic Toxicity:

1) In the patient with suspected local anesthetic toxicity, the initial step is supportive and symptomatic treatment in the form of stabilization of potential life threats, impending airway compromise, significant hypotension, and treatment of dysrhythmias and seizures so; maintain airway and respirationusing O_2 supply by face mask up to endotracheal intubation and mechanical ventilation if needed.

2) CNS manifestations, such as seizures, can be treated successfully with benzodiazepines (small increments of diazepam 2.5 mg) and barbiturates (e.g. phenobarbital) and 2 mg/kg of intravenous thiopental. Avoid use of phenytoin because it shares pharmacologic properties (i.e. sodium channel blockade) with lidocaine and may potentiate toxicity. A recent report has suggested that the intravenous injection of 100 ml of 20% lipid emulsion may have a beneficial role in aborting central nervous system manifestations of bupivacaine toxicity.

3) In the setting of local anesthetic induced cardiac toxicity, lidocaine has been used successfully in bupivacaine-induced dysrhythmias, but its additive CNS toxicity is still a major concern.. In cardiovascular collapse, the use of adrenergic drugs with α and β agonist effect (e.g. Ephedrine, epinephrine) is useful

4) Tachyarrhythmias due to toxicity of bupivacaine are probably best treated by electrical cardioversion or with bretylium rather than lidocaine.

5) In cases of refractory cardiovascular collapse caused by an overwhelming overdose of local anesthetic, Application of lipid emulsion infusion in the resuscitation of bupivacaine-induced cardiac arrest also known as "lipid rescue". The proposed mechanism is that lipid infusion accelerates the decline in bupivacaine myocardial content (reduced tissue binding) by creating a lipid phase that extracts the lipid-soluble bupivacaine molecules from the aqueous plasma phase.

12 -Role of intravenous fluids in protection against spinal induced hypotension.

12-1 Lactated Ringer's solution:

- **Physical and chemical properties**

One litre of lactated Ringer's solution contains:

- 130 mEq of sodium ion = 130 mmol/L
- 109 mEq of chloride ion = 109 mmol/L
- 28 mEq of lactate = 28 mmol/L
- 4 mEq of potassium ion = 4 mmol/L
- 3 mEq of calcium ion = 1.5 mmol/L

Lactated Ringer's has an osmolarity of 273 mOsm/L. The lactate is metabolized into bicarbonate by the liver, which can help correct metabolic acidosis. Although its pH is 6.5, it is an alkalizing solution.

The solution is formulated to have concentrations of potassium and calcium that are similar to the ionized concentrations found in normal blood plasma. To maintain electrical neutrality, the solution has a lower level of sodium than that found in isotonic saline or plasma.

12-2 colliods:

Colloid solutions, such as 5% albumin, 6% hydroxyethylstarch (HES), and gelatin, are also used for preventing the hypotension associated with spinal anesthesia . Preloading the circulation with crystalloids or colloids is aimed at the volume expansion that neutralizes the vasodilatation induced by sympathectomy due to subarachnoid blockade.

- Human albumin solution

Albumin is the principal natural colloid comprising 50 to 60% of all plasma proteins. It contributes to 80% of the normal oncotic pressure. Albumin consists of a single polypeptide chain of 585 amino acids with a molecular weight of 69,000 Dalton.

Metabolism

Albumin is synthesized only in the liver and has a half-life of approximately 20 days. After synthesis albumin is not stored but secreted into the blood stream with 42% remaining in the intravascular compartment[1].

Degree of volume expansion:

5% solution is isooncotic and leads to 80% initial volume expansion whereas 25% solution is hyperoncotic and leads to 200 - 400% increase in volume within 30 minutes. The effect persists for 16 - 24 h.

Advantages:

1. Natural colloid: As albumin is a natural colloid it is associated with lesser side-effects like pruritus, anaphylactoid reactions and coagulation abnormalities compared to synthetic colloids
2. Degree of volume expansion: 25%Albumin has a greater degree of volume expansion as compared to rest of colloids. 5% albumin solution has a similar degree of volume expansion as compared to hetastarch but greater than gelatins and dextrans.

1. Cost effectiveness: Albumin is expensive as compared to synthetic colloids.
2. Volume overload so should be used carefully in cardiac paitents ,and in patients have interstitial edema.

12-3 Dextran.

Dextrans are highly branched polysaccharide molecules which are available for use as an artificial colloid.

Physicochemical properties:

Two dextran solutions are now most widely used, a 6% solution with an average molecular weight of 70,000 (dextran 70) and a 10% solution with an average weight of 40,000 (dextran 40, low-molecular-weight dextran).

Metabolism & Excretion

Kidneys primarily excrete dextran solutions. Smaller molecules (14000–18000 kDa) are excreted in 15minutes, whereas larger molecules stay in circulation for several days. Up to 40% of dextran-40 and 70% of dextran-70 remain in circulation at 12 h.

Degree of volume expansion:

Both dextran-40 and dextran-70 lead to a higher volume expansion as compared to HES and 5% albumin. The duration lasts for 6–12 hours.

Advantages:

1. Volume expansion: Dextrans leads to 100–150% increase in intravascular volume
2. Microcirculation: Dextran 40 helps in improving microcirculatory flow by two mechanisms, i.e., by decreasing the viscosity of blood by haemodilution and by inhibiting erythrocytic aggregation.

Disadvantages:

1. Anaphylactic reactions: Dextrans cause more severe anaphylactic reactions than the gelatins or the starches. The reactions are due to dextran reactive antibodies which trigger the release of vasoactive mediators. Incidence of reactions can be reduced by pre-treatment with a hapten (Dextran 1).
2. Coagulation abnormalities: Dextrans lead to decreased platelet adhesiveness, decreased factor VIII, increased fibrinolysis and

coating of endothelium is decreased. Larger doses of dextran have been associated with significant bleeding complications.
3. Interference with cross-match: Dextrans coat the surface of red blood cells and can interfere with the ability to cross-match blood. Dextrans also increase erythrocyte sedimentation rate.
4. Precipitation of acute renal failure: A possible mechanism for this is the accumulation of the dextran molecules in the renal tubules causing tubular plugging. Renal failure following dextran use is more often reported when renal perfusion is reduced or when preexisting renal damage is present.

14-4 Hydroxyethyl starches (HES)

- Physiochemical Properties:

HES preparations are characterized by the following properties.

1. Concentration: low (6%) or high (10%).

Concentration mainly influences the initial volume effect: 6% HES solutions are iso-oncotic in vivo, with 1 l replacing about 1 l of blood loss, whereas 10% solutions are hyperoncotic, with a volume effect considerably exceeding the infused volume (about 145%).

2. Average Molecular Weight (MW): low ($\simeq$70 kDa), medium (200 kDa), or high ($\simeq$ 450 kDa).

Degree of volume expansion:

The increase in colloid osmotic pressure obtained with HES is equivalent to albumin. HES results in 100% volume expansion similar to 5% albumin. It results in greater volume expansion as compared to gelatins. Duration of volume expansion is usually 8-12 h.

Advantages:

1. Cost effectiveness: HES is less expensive as compared to albumin and is associated with a comparable volume of expansion.
2. Maximum allowable volume: Maximum volume which can be transfused of medium weight HES (130 kDa) with medium degree of substitution (0.4) is 50 ml/kg. This is greater as compared to other synthetic colloids like dextrans.

Disadvantages:

1. Coagulation: HES administration is associated with reduction in circulating factor VIII and von Willebrand factor levels, impairment of platelet function, prolongation of partial thromboplast in time and activated partial thromboplastin time and increases bleeding complications.

2. **Accumulation:** It gets deposited in various tissues including skin, liver, muscle, spleen, intestine, trophoblast and placental stroma. Such depositions have been associated with pruritus.
3. **Anaphylactoid Reactions**
4. **Renal impairment:** HMW HES has been found to be associated with increased creatinine levels, oliguria, acute renal failure in patients ill with existing renal impairment.

12-5 Third-generation HES: tetrastarch

The development of newer starch-based plasma volume expanders has been driven by a need to improve safety and pharmacological properties while maintaining the volume efficacy of previous HES generations. Reductions in MW and MS have led to products with shorter half-lives, improved pharmacokinetic and.

Safety profile of tetrastarches vis-à-vis earlier-generation HES

Effects on Coagulation and Platelet Function: A number of studies have investigated the in vitro and in vivo effects of various HES products on coagulation and platelet function. Overall, the more rapidly degradable HES products have been found to have a greatly reduced effect on the coagulation process compared to older products.

13-Crystalloid versus colloid in spinal induced hypotension:

Many studies concluded that physiologic explanation of the differences between crystalloid and colloid, at 30 minutes, only 28% of the administered lactated Ringer's solution remained in the intravascular space compared with 100% of the HES solution.
HES increases the blood volume, cardiac output, and decreases the incidence of hypotension. Colloid is a more effective volume expander because it remains longer in the intravascular compartment. However expansion of the intravascular space cannot completely abolish the risk of hypotension.

Other studies concluded that colloids may be due to decreased afterload by release of atrial natriuretic peptide as a result of stretched atrium or by reduction of arterial blood oxygen content leads to peripheral vasodilation. Prevention of central sympathetic block may may be have an important role in the prevention of post spinal hypotension.

Many studies found that HES was superior to modified gelatin but failed to offer an explanation. Important effects of prophylactic or therapeutic administration of HES colloids are the maintenance and rapid restoration of intravascular volume. Besides these effects on macrocirculation, effects on microcirculation and tissue oxygenation are important for the preservation of organ function. HES 130/0.4

(6%) was found superior regarding tissue oxygenation when compared with crystalloids in major abdominal surgery, and provided a larger and faster increase of tissue oxygen tension when compared with other HES solutions after infusion in volunteers.

14-Drugs used in spinal induced hypotension:

14-1 Epinephrine

Profound hypotension and bradycardia, which persists despite treatment, should be treated with epinephrine in a dose of 5-10 mcg IVP. Epinephrine should be repeated and/or the dose increased until the desired response is achieved.

14-2 phenylephrine,

it is a direct acting alpha adrenergic agonist, which increases venous tone and causes arterial constriction. If hypotension is associated with bradycardia, then phenylephrine should be avoided.

Phenylephrine may cause reflex bradycardia.

14-3 Ephedrine :

has a direct beta adrenergic effect, increasing heart rate and contractility as well as some indirect vasoconstriction (α). This may be a better choice in this situation.

- **Pharmacology of Ephedrine**

Description:

Ephedrine is a sympathomimetic drug, chemically designated α-[1-(methylamino) ethyl] benzenemethanol sulfate (2:1)(salt). It has the following structural formula

$$\left[\bigcirc \begin{array}{c} OH \\ | \\ C \\ | \\ H \end{array} \begin{array}{c} NHCH_3 \\ | \\ C-CH_3 \\ | \\ H \end{array} \right]_2 \cdot H_2SO_4$$

pharmacological structure of ephedrine

Obtained from plants of the genus *Ephedra*, and has been used in Chinese and eastern Indian medicine for over 5000 years. Ephedrine is just one of the alkaloids isolated from the *Ephedra spp*

- **Mechanism of Action:**

Ephedrine releases endogenous norepinephrine from its storage sites. This represents an indirect sympathomimetic effect. Norepinephrine, in turn, stimulates various alpha and beta-receptors. Ephedrine may also stimulate beta-receptors directly, particularly in bronchiolar smooth muscle. Beta-adrenergic effects result from the production of cyclic-AMP by activation of the enzyme adenylatecyclase.

- **Cardiovascular effects of Ephedrine:**
- **Contractility:**

Stimulation of $beta_1$-receptors in the heart results in positive inotropic effects which are primarily responsible for the pressor effects of the drug.

- **Heart rate:**

Although ephedrine exerts a positive chronotropic effect through the sinoatrial node, this effect can be reversed by a compensatory vagal response to the increase in blood pressure. Consequently, both sinus bradycardia and tachycardia have been observed. Some patients do not exhibit changes in heart rate. Arrhythmia can occur following high doses.

- <u>Coronary blood flow:</u>

The effects of ephedrine on coronary blood flow may be dose dependent, but in general, ephedrine usually increases coronary blood flow. This increase in blood flow may be due to the dilation of coronary arteries or as a result of an increase in blood pressure.

- <u>Systemic vascular resistance:</u>

In the periphery, ephedrine can produce both vasodilation by the stimulation of $beta_2$-receptors or vasoconstriction as a result of stimulating $alpha_1$-receptors. Constriction of arterioles in the skin, mucous membranes, and viscera occur following ephedrine administration, while vasodilation occurs in the skeletal muscle. Constriction or dilation of the pulmonary and cerebral vessels can occur. Ephedrine increases systolic and diastolic blood pressure. Pressor responses are slower but last longer than with epinephrine or norepinephrine.

- <u>Renal effects:</u>

Parenteral ephedrine decreases renal blood flow by constricting renal blood vessels. Hypotensive patients who are not hypovolemic will initially experience reduced blood and urine flow, which will increase as blood pressure returns to normal.

- **Respiratory system:**

Ephedrine relaxes bronchial smooth muscle by the stimulation of $beta_2$-receptors, relieving mild bronchospasm, improving air exchange and increasing vital capacity.

- **CNS effects:**

Ephedrine has a stimulating effect on the CNS, but less pronounced than amphetamines.

- **GIT effects:**

Ephedrine generally relaxes smooth muscle in the gastrointestinal tract, but contracts the urinary bladder trigone and sphincter, and relaxes the detrusor muscle, which can cause urinary retention.

- **Effects on the uterus:**

Effects on the uterus are variable, but when ephedrine is used to correct hypotension resulting from spinal anesthesia during delivery, it has resulted in improved uterine blood flow.

- **Effects of Epedrine on blood glucose:**

Ephedrine causes glycogenolysis, but not to the same degree as epinephrine; hyperglycemia is not likely with ephedrine. Increases in oxygen consumption and metabolic rate occur as a result of central stimulation.

- Pharmacokinetics:

    ephedrine may be crosses the placenta and distributes into breast milk. Small amounts of ephedrine are metabolized by the liver via oxidative deamination, demethylation, aromatic hydroxylation, and conjugation. Metabolites have been identified as p-hydroxyephedrine, p-hydroxynorephedrine, norephedrine and conjugates of these metabolites. Ephedrine and its metabolites are excreted primarily in the urine, mostly as unchanged drug. The elimination of ephedrine and its metabolites is enhanced by an acidic urinary pH. The elimination half-life of ephedrine is reported to be about 3 hours if the urinary pH is 5, and about 6 hours at a urinary pHof 6.5[140]

- Pharmacokinetics

    _The clinical effects of ephedrine are observed immediately following intravenous route. Ephedrine is rapidly and completely absorbed following intramuscular administration. Absorption by the intramuscular route is slightly more rapid (within 10—20 minutes) than the subcutaneous .

- **Clinical pharmacology:**

Therapeutic doses of ephedrine produce mainly relaxation of smooth muscle and, if norepinephrine stores are intact, cardiac stimulation and increased systolic and usually increased diastolic blood pressure. Its vasopressor effect results largely from increased cardiac output and to a lesser extent from peripheral vasoconstriction. Pressor responses to parenteral ephedrine are slower but more prolonged than those produced by epinephrine.

Ephedrine stimulates both alpha and beta receptors and its peripheral actions are due partly to norepinephrine release and partly to direct effect on receptors. Ephedrine may deplete norepinephrine stores in sympathetic nerve endings, so that tachyphylaxis to cardiac and pressor effects of the drug may develop.

Glycogenolysis in the liver is increased by ephedrine but not as much as by epinephrine; usual doses of ephedrine are unlikely to produce hyperglycemia.

Ephedrine is rapidly and completely absorbed following parenteral injection. Pressor and cardiac responses to ephedrine persist for one hour following intramuscular or subcutaneous administration of 25 to 50 mg.

- **Sides effects of Ephedrine:**

- <u>Cardiovascular:</u>tachycardia, cardiac arrhythmias, angina pectoris, vasoconstriction with hypertension
- <u>Dermatological</u>: flushing, sweating, acne vulgaris
- <u>Gastrointestinal</u>: nausea
- <u>Genitourinary</u>: decreased urination due to vasoconstriction of renal arteries. Also, difficulty urinating is not uncommon, as alpha-agonists such as ephedrine constrict the internal urethral sphincter, mimicking the effects of sympathetic nervous system stimulation.
- <u>Nervous system</u>: restlessness, confusion, insomnia, mild euphoria, mania/hallucinations (rare except in previously existing psychiatric conditions), delusions, formication (may be possible, but lacks documented evidence) paranoia, hostility, panic, agitation
- <u>Respiratory</u>: dyspnea, pulmonary edema
- <u>Miscellaneous</u>: dizziness, headache, tremor, hyperglycemic reactions, dry mouth

- **Contraindications:**

1-Closed angle glaucoma

2-Concomitant or recent use(previous14 days) of MAO inhibitors

3-Pheochromocytoma

4-Idiopathic hypertrophic subaortic stenosis

5-Tachyarrhythmias or ventricular fibrillation

6-Hypersensitivity to ephedrine

- **Ephedrine during pregnancy:**

Ephedrine-like drugs are teratogenic in some animal species, but human teratogenicity has not been suspected .Ephedrine has been assigned to pregnancy category C by the FDA.

- **Ephedrine and spinal anesthesia:**

Ephedrine is routinely used to treat or prevent maternal hypotension following spinal anesthesia .Significant increases in fetal heart rate and beat-to-beat variability may occur, but these effects may have been the result of normal reflexes following hypotension-associated bradycardias. A recent study, however, has demonstrated the placental passage of ephedrine with fetal levels at delivery approximately 70% of the maternal concentration. The presence of ephedrine in the fetal circulation is probably a major cause of the fetal heart rate changes.

- **Ephedrine in lactating mothers:**

Ephedrine is excreted into human milk. Breast-feeding is considered to be contraindicated by the manufacturer.

A single case report has been located describing adverse effects in a 3-month-old nursing infant of a mother consuming a long-acting preparation containing 120 mg of d-isoephedrine and 6 mg of dexbrompheniramine . The mother had begun taking the preparation on a twice-daily schedule 1 or 2 days prior to onset of the infant's symptoms. The infant exhibited irritability, excessive crying, and disturbed sleeping patterns that resolved spontaneously within 12 hours when breast feeding was stopped.

14-4-Ondansetron:

The molecular formula is C18H19N3O•HCl•2H2O, representing a molecular weight of 365.9. Ondansetron hydrochloride USP (dihydrate) is a white to off-white powder that is soluble in water and normal saline.

Ondansetron tablets, USP for oral administration contain Ondansetron hydrochloride USP (dihydrate) equivalent to 4 mg or 8 mg of Ondansetron. Each film-coated tablet also contains the inactive ingredients anhydrous lactose, microcrystalline cellulose, pregelatinized starch (maize), magnesium stearate, triacetin, titanium dioxide and hypromellose. In addition 8 mg tablet also contains iron oxide yellow.

- *Ondansetron - Clinical Pharmacology*
- **Pharmacodynamics**
  Ondansetron is a selective 5-HT3 receptor antagonist. While its mechanism of action has not been fully characterized, Ondansetron is not a dopamine-receptor antagonist. Serotonin receptors of the 5-HT3 type are

present both peripherally on vagal nerve terminals and centrally in the chemoreceptor trigger zone of the area postrema. It is not certain whether Ondansetron's antiemetic action is mediated centrally, peripherally, or in both sites. However, cytotoxic chemotherapy appears to be associated with release of serotonin from the enterochromaffin cells of the small intestine. In humans, urinary 5-HIAA (5-hydroxyindoleacetic acid) excretion increases after cisplatin administration in parallel with the onset of emesis. The released serotonin may stimulate the vagal afferents through the 5-HT3 receptors and initiate the vomiting reflex.

- *.Pharmacokinetics:*

Ondansetron is well absorbed from the gastrointestinal tract and undergoes some first-pass metabolism. Mean bioavailability in healthy subjects, following administration of a single 8 mg tablet, is approximately 56%.

Ondansetron is extensively metabolized in humans, with approximately 5% of a radiolabeled dose recovered as the parent compound from the urine. The primary metabolic pathway is hydroxylation on the indole ring followed by subsequent glucuronide or sulfate conjugation. Although some nonconjugated metabolites have pharmacologic activity, these are not found plasma at concentrations likely to significantly contribute to the biological activity of Ondansetron.

13-Role of pharmacologic agents prevention of hypotension:
Prophylactic administration of vasopressors may be more effective than prehydration . α-Adrenergic agonists (phenylephrine) reliably increase arterial blood pressure by increasing systemic vascular resistance; but the heart rate and cardiac output may decrease because of increased afterload . Many studies have shown that phenylephrine does not harm the fetus when given in the dose range required to prevent hypotension. There is no Evidence for the observation that phenylephrine depress fetal pH and base excess than ephedrine. And the controversies remain.

Mixed α- and β-adrenergic agents (ephedrine) are also effective for increasing arterial blood pressure and preventing hypotension but act by primarily increasing heart rate and cardiac output with a smaller increase in systemic vascular resistance .

Previous studies found that ephedrine is the better vasopressor for hypotension with spinal anesthesia in the parturient because it maintains uteroplacental blood flow. Ephedrine's action is mainly indirect, via stimulating release of norepinephrine from sympathetic nerve terminals; and there is no direct sympathetic innervations to the uteroplacental circulation ,so it is relatively resistant to the vasoconstrictive effects of ephedrine . IM ephedrine is difficult to predict both absorption and peak effect , and also observed reactive hypertension, particularly if spinal anesthesia was unsuccessful. Prophylactic Ephedrine infusion or bolus doses administered has been considered the ideal routes for preventing hypotension for .The effect of an .IV bolus of ephedrine on arterial pressure is transient and it lasts for only 10 – 15 min .So ephedrine infusion is considered to prevent spinal-induced hypotension

ephedrine increases uteroplacental blood flow however there is evidence of increased fetal acidosis associated with use of ephedrine, The most accepted explanation is that ephedrine increase metabolic rate of the fetus, A study by Cooper et al.2002 used an index to assess where the umbilical artery acidosis was occurring. They compare pCO_2 of the umbilical artery and the pCO_2 of the umbilical vein. They found that if there is increase in Co_2 level, so acidosis was being generated in the fetus. They found that umbilical artery pCO_2 minus umbilical vein pCO_2 in the ephedrine group correlate with a low umbilical artery pH. They also found that this index was correlated with ephedrine dose. These data are highly suggestive that ephedrine is increasing the metabolic rate of the fetus.

The reason why ephedrine depresses fetal acid–base status more than phenylephrine is controversial. Ngan Kee et al. study found that ephedrine crosses the placenta more readily than phenylephrine. This was associated with greater fetal concentrations of lactate, glucose and catecholamines, this metabolic effects secondary to stimulation of fetal beta-adrenergic receptors cause base excess with ephedrine, and thus depressed fetal pH.

The use of a lower dose aims to decrease maternal side effects (hypotension, nausea, vomiting).

- Role of onandestron in spinal induced hypotension:

Serotonin in response to decreased blood volume activates Chemoreceptors . Serotonin is released from activated thrombocytes. Serotonin Activate 5-HT3 receptors, which are G protein coupled, ligand-gated fast-ion channels, results in increased efferent vagal nerve activity, frequently producing bradycardia . Mechanoreceptors in the heart wall that trigger the BJR, participate in systemic responses to hyper- and hypo-volaemia. In response to hypovolaemia, stimulation of cardiac sensory receptors in the left ventricle induces the BJR and results in reflex bradycardia, vasodilation and hypotension.

Many studies found that ondansetron prevented the serotonin-induced BJR, suppressed venodilatation, increased venous return to the heart and resulted in less reductions in Systolic and mean blood pressure.

Other studies found that, administration of two different doses of intravenous ondansetron, 6 mg and 12 mg, decreased spinal induced hypotension, bradycardia and shivering in comparison with saline group. .

In some anesthesia unites use an aesthetic protocol that provides for the administration 500 ml of colloid (Voluven) and ondansetron 8 mg before subarachnoid anaesthesia in elective Caesarean section, to avoid the use of ephedrine and decrease the risk of fetal acidosis.

15 -References:

1. Hawkins JL, Chang J, Palmer SK, et al. Anesthesia-related maternal mortality in the United States: 1979-2002. ObstetGynecol 2011; 117:69

2. Bucklin BA, Hawkins JL, Anderson JR, Ullrich FA. Obstetric anesthesia workforce survey: twenty-year update. Anesthesiology 2005; 103:645

3. Park GE, Hauch MA, Curlin F, Datta S, Bader AM. The effects of varying volumes of crystalloid administration before cesarean delivery on maternal hemodynamics and colloid osmotic pressure.AnesthAnalg. 1996;83:299–303.

4. Cheun JK, Kim AR. Intrathecalmeperidine as the sole agent for cesarean section. J Korean Med Sci. 1989;4:135–138.

5. Hawkins JL, Arens JF, Bucklin BA, et al. Practice Guidelines for Obstetric Anesthesia: An Updated Report by the American Society of Anesthesiologists Task Force on Obstetric Anesthesia.

Anesthesiology. April 2007;106(4).

6. Gerges FJ, Kanazi GE, Jabbour-khoury SI. Anesthesia for laparoscopy: a review. Journal of Clinical Anesthesia. Feb 2006;18(1).

7. Hossain N, Tayab S, Mahmood T. Spinal anaesthesia for caesarean section. J Surg Pak 2002; 7: 19-21

8. Ismail S, Huda A... An observational study of anaesthesia and surgical time in elective caesarean section: spinal compared with general anaesthesia. Int J ObstetAnesth. 2009 Oct;18(4):352-5

9. Campbell J, Sultan P. Regional anaesthesia for caesarean section: a choice of three techniques. Br J Hosp Med (Lond). 2009 Oct;70(10):605

10. Kuczkopwski KM, Reisner LS, Lin D. Anesthesia for cesarean section. In:Chestnut DH, Polley LS, Tsen LC, Wong CA, editors. Chestnut's ObstetricAnesthesia: Principles and Practice. 4th ed. Philadelphia: Mosby; 2009. p. 422-5.

11. Carvalho B, Coleman L, Saxena A, Fuller AJ, Riley ET. Analgesic requirements and postoperative recovery after scheduled compared to unplanned cesarean delivery: a retrospective chart review. Int J ObstetAnesth. 2010 Jan;19(1):10-5

12. Klohr S, Roth R, Hofmann T, Rossaint R, Heesen M. Definitions of hypotension after spinal anaesthesia for caesarean section: Literature search and applicationto parturients. ActaAnaesthesiolScand 2010;54:909-21

13. Allen TK, Muir HA, George RB, Habib AS.A survey of the management of spinal-induced hypotension for scheduled cesarean delivery. Int J ObstetAnesth. 2009 Oct;18(4):356-61.

14. Kinsella SM. A prospective audit of regional anaesthesia failure in 5080 Caesarean sections.Anaesthesia. 2008 Aug;63(8):822-32. Epub 2008 Jun 28

15. Greene NM. The physiology of spinal anesthesia. 3rd ed. Baltimore: Williams and Wilkins, 1981.

16. Moore DC, Bridenbaugh LD. Spinal block. a review of 11,574 cases. JAMA 1966;195:907-12.

17. Carpenter RL, Caplan RA, Brown DL, et al. Incidence and risk factors for side effects of spinal anesthesia. Anesthesiology 1992;

18. Clark SL, Cotton DB, Pivarnik JM, Lee W, Hankins GD, Benedetti TJ, Phelan JP. Position change and central hemodynamic profile during normal third-trimester pregnancy and post partum. Am J Obstet Gynecol. 1991;164:883–887.

19. Cyna AM, Andrew M, Emmett RS, Middleton P, Simmons SW. Techniques for preventing hypotension during spinal anaesthesia for caesarean section. Cochrane Database Syst Rev 2006;18(4)

20. Bhagat H, Malohtra K, Ghildyal SK, Srivastava PC. Evaluation of preloading and vasoconstrictors as a combined prophylaxis for hypotension during subarachnoid anaesthesia. Indian J Anaesth 2004; 48 (4): 299-303

21. Higuchi H, Hirata J, Adachi Y, Kazama T. Influence of lumbosacral cerebrospinal fluid density, velocity, and volume on extent and duration of plain bupivacaine spinal anesthesia. Anesthesiology 2004;100:106–14

22. Carpenter RL, Caplan RA, Brown DL, Stephenson C, Wu R. Incidence and Risk Factors for Side Effects of Spinal Anaesthesia. Anaesthesiology1992;76(6)906-916

23. Arndt JO, Bömer W, Krauth J, Marquardt B. Incidence and time course of cardiovascular side effects during spinal anaesthesia after prophylactic administration of intravenous fluids or

vasoconstrictors. Anesth Analg 1998; 87 (2): 347-354

24. Rooke GA, Freund PR, Jacobson AF. Hemodynamic response and change in organ blood volume during spinal anesthesia in elderly men with cardiac disease. Anesth Analg 1997; 85 (1): 99-105

25. Butterworth J. Physiology of spinal anesthesia: What are the implications for management? Reg Anesth Pain Med 1998; 23 (4): 370-373

26. Brooker RF, Butterworth JFT, Kitzman DW, Berman JM, Kashtan HI, McKinley AC. Treatment of hypotension after hyperbaric tetracaine spinal anesthesia: A randomized, double-blind, cross-over comparison of phenylephrine and epinephrine. Anesthesiology1997;86(4):797-805

27. Critchley LA, Conway F. Hypotension during subarachnoid anaesthesia: haemodynamic effects of colloid and metaraminol. Br J Anaesth1996;76(5):734-736

28. Lovstad RZ, Granhus G, Hetland S. Bradycardia and asystolic cardiac arrest during spinal anaesthesia: A report of five cases. Acta

Anaesthsiol,Scand,2000;44(1):48-52

29. WollmanSB, marx GE; acute hydration for prevention of hypotension of spinal anaesthesia in parturients. Anaesthesiology 1968;29:374-80.

30. JacksonR, reid JA, thorburn j. volume preload is not essential to prevent spinal induced hypotension at cesarean section. british Journal of anaesthesiology 1995;75:262-5

31. RoutCC, Rocke DA. Prophylactic intramuscular ephedrine prior to cesarean section. Anaesthesia and intensive care1992;20:448.52

32. Kang YG, Abouleish E, Caritis S. Prophylactic intravenous ephedrine infusion during spinal anesthesia for Cesarean section. AnesthAnalg 1983;61:83942

33. Rout CC, Rocke DA, Levin J et al. — A reevaluation of the role of crystalloid preload in the prevention of hypotension associated with spinal anesthesia for elective cesarean section. Anesthesiology, 1993;79:262-269.

34. Ralston DH, Shnider SM, DeLorimier AA — Effects of equipotent ephedrine, metaraminol, mephentermine, and methoxamine on uterine blood flow in the pregnant ewe. Anesthesiology, 1974; 40:354-370.

35. Karinine J, Rasanen J, Alahuhta S, Joupilla P .Maternal and uteroplacental hemodynamic state in preeclamptiv patients during spinal anaesthesia for caesarean section .Br J Anaesth. 1996 May ;76(5):616-20.

36. Capeless EL, Clapp JR. Cardiovascular changes in the early stages of pregnancy. Am J ObstetGynecol 1989; 161:1439.

37. Duvekot JJ, Peeters LL. Maternal cardiovascular hemodynamic adaptation to pregnancy. ObstetGynecolSurv 1994; 49(12 Suppl):S1.

38. Widerhorn J, Widerhorn AL, Rahimtoola SH, et al. WPW syndrome during pregnancy: Increased incidence of supraventricular arrhythmias. Am Heart J 1992; 123:796.

39. Thompson LP and Weiner CP , estadiol effect and nitric oxide synthase activity. Circulation.1997 ; 95:709–714.

40. Lees MM, Taylor SH, Scott DB, et al. A study of cardiac output at rest throughout pregnancy.Am J ObstetGynecol BrCommonw 1967; 74:319.

41. Ueland K, Novy MJ, Peterson EN, et al. Maternal cardiovascular dynamics. Part IV. The influence of gestational age on the maternal cardiovascular response to posture and exercise.Am J ObstetGynecol 1969; 104:856.

42. Marx GF. Aortocaval compression; incidence and prevention. Bull NY Acad Med 1974; 50:443.

43. Cole PL, St. John Sutton M. Normal cardiopulmonary adjustments to pregnancy: Cardiovascular evaluation. CardiovascClin 1989; 19:37.

44..Bhagwat AR, Engel PJ. Heart disease and pregnancy.CardiolClin 1995; 13:163.

45..Theunissen I, Parer J. Fluid and electrolytes in pregnancy. ClinObstetGynecol1994; 37:3-15.

46.. Conklin KA. Maternal physiological adaptations during gestation, labor and the puerperium.SeminAnesth 1991; 10:221-234.

47.. Sharma SK, Philip J, Wiley J. Thromboelastographic changes in healthy parturients and postpartum women. AnesthAnalg1997; 85:94.

48. ACOG. Practice bulletin no. 125: chronic hypertension in pregnancy. Obstet Gynecol. Feb 2012;119(2 Pt 1):396

49.Landesman R, Holze W, Scherr L. Fetal mortality in essential hyper- tension. ObstetGynecol 1955;6:354-65.

50. Tygart SG, McRoyan DK, Spinnato JA, et al. Longitudinal studies of platelet indices during normal pregnancy. Am J ObstetGynecol1986;

154:883-887.

51..Lottan M, Mashiach R, Namestnikov M. Hematologic diseases. In: Birnbach DJ, Gatt SP, Datta S, ed. Textbook of Obstetric Anesthesia, New York: Churchill Livingstone; 2000:586-596.

52.. Ross A. Physiologic changes of pregnancy. In: Birnbach DJ, Gatt SP, Datta S, ed. Textbook of Obstetric Anesthesia, New York: Churchill Livingstone; 2000:31-45.

53. Chadwick HS, Posner K, Caplan R, et al , A comparison of obstetric and non-obstetric anesthesia malpractice claims. Anesthesiology.2001 ;74(2):242-9.

54. Camaan WR and OstheimerGW , Physiological adaptations during pregnancy. IntAnesthesiolClin.2001 ;28(1):2-10.

55.Sandhar BK, Elliot RH, Windram I, et al. Peripartum changes in gastric emptying. Anaesthesia 1992; 47:196.

56..Sibai BM, Frangieh A. Maternal adaptation to pregnancy. CurrOpinObstetGynecol 1995; 7:420.

57..Kiserud T, Acharya G (2004). "The fetal circulation".Prenatal Diagnosis24 (13): 1049–1059

58. Valdes G, Kaufmann P, Corthorn J, et al. Vasodilator factors in the systemic and local adaptations to

pregnancy. ReprodBiolEndocrinol 2009; 7:79.

59.. Rosenfeld CR, Naden RP. Responses of uterine and nonuterine tissues to angiotensin II in ovine pregnancy. Am J Physiol 1995; 257:H17.

60. Reynolds LP, Borowicz PP, Caton JS, et al.Uteroplacental vascular development and placental function: an update. Int J DevBiol 2010; 54:355.

61. Ramesar SV, Mackraj I , Gathiram P , Moodley J. Sildenafil citrate improves fetal outcomes in pregnant, L-NAME treated, Sprague-Dawley rats. Eur J ObstetGynecolReprodBiol 2010; 149:22.

62. Rudolph AM, Heymann MA. Circulatory changes during growth in the fetal lamb. Circ Res 1970; 26:289.

63. Thaete LG , Dewey ER , Neerhof MG. Endothelin and the regulation of uterine and placental perfusion in hypoxia-induced fetal growth restriction. J SocGynecolInvestig 2004; 11:16.

64. Brown Jr WU, Bell GC, Alper MH. Acidosis, local anesthetics and the newborn.ObstetGynecol1976; 48:27-30.

65. Drasner K, Larson MD: Spinal and epidural anesthesia. In: Basics of anesthesia. Robert K. Stoeling, Ronald D.Miller (eds). Fifth edtion, 2007;242-246.

66. Bernard CM: Management of anaethesia. Epidural and spinal anaesthesia. In: textbook of clinical anaesthesia. Barash PG, Cullen BF, Stoeling RK (eds). Fifth edition, 2005; 645-668. Philadelphia. Lippincott Williams & Wilkins.

67. Bridenbaugh PO, Greene NM: Spinal (subarachnoid) neural blockade. In: neural blockade in clinical anaethesia and Management of Pain. cousinsMJ, Bridenbaugh PO (eds). Third edition, 1998;203-241. Philadelphia. Lippincott-raven.

68. Drasner K: Subarachnoid. In: Regional Anaesthesia. Atlas of anatomy and technique. Hahn MB, McQuillan PM, Sheplock GJ (eds). 2005; 221-229. St. Louis. Mosby.

69. Butterworth J, Piccione W, Berrizbeitia L et al: Augmentation of venous return by adrenergic agonists during spinal anesthesia. AnesthAnalg 1986,65:612

70. Carpenter RL, Caplan RA, Brown DL et al: Incidence and risk factors for side effect of spinal anaesthesia. Anaesthesiology 1992,76:906

71. Phero JC, Bridenbaugh PO, Edstrom HH et al: Hypotension in spinal anesthesia: A comparison of isobaric tetracaine with epinephrine and isobaric bupivacaine without epinephrine. AnesthAnalg 1987,66:549

72. Venn PJ, Simpson DA, Rubin AP, Edstrom HH: Effect of fluid preloading on cardiovascular variables after spinal anaesthesia with glaucose-free 0.75% bupivacaine. Br J Anaeth 1989,63:682.

73. Marhofer P, Faryniak B, Oismuller C et al: Cardiovascular effects of 6% hetastarch and lactated Ringer's solution during spinal anesthesia .Reg.Anesth Pain Med 1999, 24(5):399

74. Greene NM: Perspectives in spinal anesthesia. RegAnesth 7:55, 1982.

75. Tarkkila P, Isola J: A regression model for identifying patients at high risk of hypotension, bradycardia and nausea during spinal anesthesia. ActaAnesthesiol Scand1992, 36:554

76. Halpern SH and Chochinov M.The use of vasopressors for the prevention and treatment of hypotension secondary to regional anesthesia for cesarean section.Oxford.Evidence based obstetric anesthesia. 2005; 101–07.

77. Breen TW, cardiac arrest during regional anesthesia. Evidence-based obstetric anesthesia.Massachusets,USA.2003;2:123–28.

78. Spence AG Lipid reversal of central nervous system symptoms of bupivacaine toxicity. Anesthesiology; 2007, 107 (3): 516-517.

79. May CS, Pickup ME, Paterson JW. The acute and chronic bronchodilator effects of ephedrine in asthmatic patients. Br J

ClinPharmacol. 1975 Dec;2(6):533–537

80. Wilkinson GR, Beckett AH. Absorption, metabolism, and excretion of the ephedrines in man. II. Pharmacokinetics. J Pharm Sci. 1968 Riegelman S, Loo JC, Rowland M. Shortcomings in pharmacokinetic analysis by conceiving the body to exhibit properties of a single compartment. J Pharm Sci. 1968 Jan;57(1):117–123.

81. Rowland M. Influence of route of administration on drug availability. J Pharm Sci. 1972 Jan;61(1):70–74.

82. Bedford laboratories . Ephedrine sulphate injection, USP(50mg/ml) prescribing information . Bedford.OH;1998Aug.

83. Gurley BJ, Grdner SF .White LM et al. Ephedrine pharmacokinetics after ingestion of nutritional supplements containing Ephedra sinica (ma huang).TherDrugMonit.1998;20;439-45(IDIDS 411627).

84. MaynePharma. Ephedrine sulfate injection DBL (Approved Product Information). Melbourne: MaynePharma; 2004

85. Nishimura H, Tanimura T. Clinical Aspects of The Teratogenicity of Drugs. New York, NY:American Elsevier, 1976:231168.Shepard TH.Catalog of Teratogenic Agents. 3rd ed. Baltimore, MD:Johns Hopkins University Press, 1980:1345

86. Williams EL, Hildebrand KL, McCormick SA, Bedel MJ (May

1999)."The effect of intravenous lactated Ringer's solution versus 0.9% sodium chloride solution on serum osmolality in human volunteers". Anesth.Analg.88 (5): 999–1003.

87. Sharma SK, Gajraj NM, Sidawi JE. Prevention of hypotension during spinal anesthesia: A comparison of intravascular administration of hetastarch versus lactated Ringer's solution. Anesth Analg 1997; 84 (1): 111-114

88. Buggy D, Higgins P, Moran C, O'Brien D, O'Donovan F, McCarroll M. Prevention of spinal anesthesia-induced hypotension in the elderly: Comparison between preanesthetic administration of crystalloids, colloids, and no prehydration. Anesth Analg 1997; 84 (1): 106-110

89. Ueyama H, Yan-Ling H, Tanigami H, Mashimo T, Yoshiya I. Effects of crystalloid and colloid preload on blood volume in the parturient undergoing spinal anesthesia for elective Cesarean section. Anesthesiology 1999; 91 (6): 1571-1576

90. Rout C, Rocke DA. Spinal hypotension associated with Cesarean section. Will preload ever work? Anesthesiology 1999; 91 (6): 1565-1567

91. Allen TK, Muir HA, George RB, Habib AS. A survey of the management of spinal-induced hypotension for scheduled cesarean

delivery. Int J Obstet Anesth 2009; 18 (4): 356-361.

92. Madi-Jebara S, Ghosn A, Sleilaty G, et al. Prevention of hypotension after spinal anesthesia for cesarean section: 6% hydroxyethyl starch 130/0.4 (Voluven) versus lactated Ringer's solution. J Med Liban 2008; 56 (4): 203-207.

93. Tamilselvan P, Fernando R, Bray J, et al. The effects of crystalloid and colloid preload on cardiac output in the parturient undergoing planned caesarean delivery under spinal anaesthesia: a randomized trial. Anesth Analg 2009; 109 (6): 1916-1921.

94. Marthru M, Rao TL, Kartha RK, Shanmugham M, Jacobs HK. Intravenous albumin administration for prevention of spinal hypotension during caesarean section. Anesth Analg 1980; 59 (9): 655-658

95. Baraka AS, Taha SK, Ghabach MB, Sibaii AA, Nader AM. Intravascular administration of polymerized gelatin versus isotonic saline for prevention of spinal-induced hypotension. Anesth Analg 1994; 78 (2): 301-305

96. Karinen J, Rasanen J, Alahuhta S, et al. Effect of crystalloid and colloid preloading on uteroplacental and maternal haemodynamic state during spinal anaesthesia for caesarean section. Br J Anaesth 1995; 75 (5): 531-535

97. Riley E, Cohen S, Rubenstein A, Flanagan B. Prevention of hypotension after spinal anaesthesia for caesarean section: six percent hetastarch versus lactated Ringer's solution. Anesth Analg 1995; 81(4): 838-42

98. Vercauteren M, Hoffmann V, Steenberge AV, Adriaensen H. Hydroxyethylstarch compared with modified gelatin as volume preload before spinal anaesthesia for Caesarean section. Br J Anaesth 1996. 76 (5): 731-733.

99. Chan WS, Irwin MG, Tong WN, Lam YH. Prevention of hypotension during spinal anaesthesia for caesarean section: Ephedrine infusion versus fluid preload. Anaesthesia 1997; 52 (9): 908-913

100. Buggy DJ, Power CK, Meeke R, O'Callaghan S, Moran C, O'Brien GT. Prevention of spinal anaesthesia-induced hypotension in the elderly: i.m. methoxamine or combined hetastarch and crystalloid. Br J Anaesth 1998; 80 (2): 199-203

101. Warwick D, Ngan Kee WD. Prevention of maternal hypotension after regional anaesthesia for caesarean section. Current Opinion in Anaesthesiology 2010; 23 (3): 304-309

102. Ngan Kee WD, Khaw KS, Tan PE, et al. Placental transfer and fetal metabolic effects of phenylephrine and ephedrine during spinal anesthesia for caesarean delivery. Anaesthesiology 2009; 111 (3): 506-512.

103. Lee A, Ngan Kee WD, Gin T. Prophylactic ephedrine prevents

hypotension during spinal anaesthesia for Caesarean delivery but does not improve neonatal outcome: a quantitative systematic review. Can J Anesth2002; 49 (6): 588-599

104. Cyna AM, Andrew M, Emmett RS, Middleton P, Simmons SW. Techniques for preventing hypotension during spinal anaesthesia for caesarean section (Review). Copyright © 2010 The Cochrane Collaboration. Published by John Wiley & Sons, Ltd.

105. Somboonviboon W, Kyokong O, Charuluxananan S, et al. Incidence and risk factors of hypotension and bradycardia after spinal anesthesia for caesarean section. J Med Assoc Thai 2008; 91 (2): 18

106. Mark AL. The Bezold-Jarisch reflex revisited: clinical implications of inhibitory reflexes originating in the heart. J Am Coll Cardiol 1983; 1 (1): 90-102

107. Aviado DM, Guevara Aviado D. The Bezold-Jarisch reflex: a historical perspective of cardiopulmonary reflexes. Ann N Y Acad Sci. 2001; 940 (6): 48-58

108. Campagna JA, Cartner C. Clinical relevance of Bezold Jarisch reflex. Anesthesiology. 2003; 98 (5): 1250-1260

109. Kaye AD, Kucera IJ. Intravascular fluid and electrolyte physiology. In: Miller RD, editor.Miller's Anesthesia. 6th edition.

Philadelphia: Churchill Livingstone; 2005. pp. 1763–98.

110. Martino P, editor. The ICU Book. 3rd edition. Philadelphia: Churchill Livingstone; 2007. Colloid and crystalloid resuscitation; pp. 233–54.

111. Dubois MJ, Vincent JL. Colloid Fluids. In: Hahn RG, Prough DS, Svensen CH, editors.Perioperative Fluid Therapy. 1st edition. New York: Wiley; 2007. pp. 153–611.

112. Linder P, Ickx B. The effects of colloid solutions on hemostasis. Can J Anesth.2006;53:30–s39.

113. Joseph S, Park G. Properties and use of albumin. In: Webb AR, editor. Intravenous Fluid Therapy, Chapter 5, Therapeutics. Germany: B. Brawn Medical Ltd; 2003.

114. Barron ME, Wilkes, Navickis RJ. A systematic review of the comparative safety of colloids. Arch Surg. 2004;139:552–563. [PubMed]

115. Yacobu A, Stoll RG, Sum CY. Pharmacokinetics of hydroxyethyl starch in normal subjects. J Clin Pharmacol. 1982;22:206–12. [PubMed]

116. Solanke TF, Khwaja MS, Kadomemu EL. Plasma volume studies with four different plasma volume expanders. J Surg Res. 1971;11:140–43. [PubMed]

117. Mydlow P, et al. Effect of enzyme inducers on Ondansetron (OND) metabolism in humans. Clin Pharmacol Ther. 1997;61:228

118. Owczuk R, Wenski W, Polak-Krzeminska A, Twardowski P, Arszułowicz R, et al. Ondansetron Given Intravenously Attenuates Arterial Blood Pressure Drop Due to Spinal Anesthesia: A Double-Blind, Placebo-Controlled Study. Regional Anesthesia & Pain Medicine 2008; 33 (4): 332-339

119. Kansal A, Mohta M, Sethi AK, Tyagi A, Kumar P. Randomised trial of intravenous infusion of ephedrine or mephentermine for management of hypotension during spinal anaesthesia for caesarean section. Anaesthesia 2005;60:28-34.

120. Cooper DW, Carpenter M, Mowbray P, Desira WR, Ryall DM, Kokri MS. Fetal and maternal effects of phenylepherine and ephedrine during spinal anaesthesia for cesarean delivery. Anesthesiology 2002;97:1582-90

121. Ngan Kee WD, Khaw KS, Ng FF, Lee BB. Prophylactic phenylepherine infusion for preventing hypotension during spinal anaesthesia for cesarean delivery. Anesth Analg 2004;98:815-21.

122. Ngan Kee WD, Khaw KS, Ng FF. Prevention of hypotension during spinal anesthesia for cesarean delivery. An effective technique using combination phenylepherine infusion and crystalloid co-hydration. Anesthesiology 2005;103:744-50.

123. Nagan Kee WD, Khaw KS, Lee BB, Lau TK, Gin T. A dose response study of prophylactic intravenous ephedrine for the prevention of hypotension during spinal anaesthesia for cesarean delivery. Anesth Analg 2000;90:1390-5.

124. Sahoo T, SenDasgupta C, Goswami A, Hazra A. Reduction in spinal-induced hypotension with ondansetron in parturients undergoing caesarean section: A double-blind randomised, placebo-controlled study. Int J of Obstetric Anasth 2012; 21 (1): 24-28

125. Tsen L. Anaesthesia for caesarean delivery. In Chesnutt DH, ed. Obstetric Anaesthesia: Principles and Practice. Philadelphia: Elsevier Mosby, 2009; 26: 521-73

126. S Palmese, M Manzi, V Visciano, A Scibilia, A Natale. Reduced Hypotension After Subarachnoid Anaesthesia With Ondansetron Most Colloids In Parturients Undergoing Caesarean Section. A Retrospective Study.. The Internet Journal of Anesthesiology. 2012 Volume 30 Number 4.

www.ingramcontent.com/pod-product-compliance
Lightning Source LLC
Chambersburg PA
CBHW051734170526
45167CB00002B/936